MUSINGS of a THERAPIST

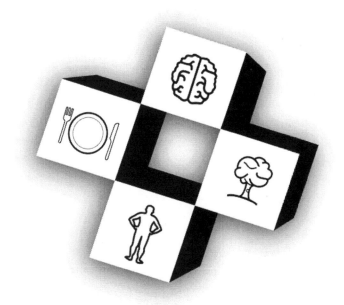

DAVE RICHES

Musings of a Therapist

© 2013, Dave Riches

ALL RIGHTS RESERVED. This book contains material protected under International and Federal Copyright Laws and Treaties. Any unauthorized reprint or use of this material is prohibited. No part of this book may be reproduced or transmitted in any form or by any means, electronic or mechanical, including photocopying, recording, or by any information storage and retrieval system without express written permission from the author.

Table of Contents

Introduction 1

Who Am I? 3

Section 1: Practicalities of Being a Therapist 8

Introduction 9

Business Plan - Can I afford to be a Therapist 11

How much should I charge? 14

What's my Brand? 18

Advertising 24

Get out and about 28

Where to Practise? 30

Note Taking 34

Section 2: A Therapist Model 37

Introduction 38

Physical Wellbeing 41

Mental Wellbeing 42

Inner Wellbeing - Nutrition 43

Environment	46
An Example	48
Section 3: Musings	**52**
Why Won't They Lie Still and Stop Talking?	53
Helping the Client to see Progress	56
Your Posture	66
Towel Management	70
Too Many Tools	75
Case Study Creation	76
Section 4: And Finally…	**79**
Bibliography	80

Introduction

Welcome. I thought it prudent to tell you what to expect from this book before you get started, so you can decide to carry on!

The purpose of this handbook, primer, hints and tips, whatever you want to call it, is to provide some advice and guidance to those starting out in the field of complementary therapies. But those of you who are more experienced might find some of the musings of interest. Of course, just like any advice, you can decide to just ignore it or take it on board as you wish.

Whilst I do mention the Bowen Technique several times, I don't think this handbook is just for Bowen practitioners. I've divided my book into three sections:

- One for the more mundane aspects of running a business;
- A section on my "model" for a complementary therapist;
- And lastly, a set of musings or anecdotes that are there to open up different pathways of thinking or progress.

Above all, I hope it generates more questions or disagreements, after all, without disagreement we get no progress, and life would soon be dull, boring, and even extinct! And if you are moved to ask me questions, point out errors or just say "I liked it" then feel free to email me at:

dave.riches@bowen-technique.co.uk.

Dave Riches
M.Sc. C.Eng., CITP, MBCS,
NLP Practitioner,
Bowen Therapist.

Musings of a Therapist

Who Am I?

Before we get into the book proper, I decided that it would be useful to have a little understanding of my background and my experiences that have shaped my thoughts about complementary therapy today. Nothing heavy, just a little light reading, but feel free to skip it at any time.

I've practised Judo since I was 8 years old and, as is the case with such a physical activity, have had my fair share of injuries. Some of them resolved by themselves, and some of them needed treatment…but no surgery thankfully. I've had many conventional and complementary treatments, all of which worked to some extent but never sorted the whole problem. As well as providing me with an understanding of injuries, and how to resolve and rehabilitate them; Judo has also provided me with an insight into balance, motion, the forces at play in movement, and an appreciation of the importance of mental focus and well-being.

My first proper introduction to complementary therapies occurred when I inflamed my rotator cuff and ended up with a frozen shoulder. On that occasion I was told that I had crystallisation in the muscles, which needed to be broken down and then followed by a set of stretches for 2 weeks. Well, I could cope with the short time of 2 weeks and the pain of the therapist breaking down the crystals didn't last too long either. So I stuck religiously to the stretching and sure enough I was back on the mat in a few weeks. Much better than the cortisone injections I'd had previously.

My next serious problem was when I popped my left collar bone on the shoulder side (acromioclavicular joint). The x-ray showed an impressive distance between the collar bone and where it should be! The doctor had no advice other than to tell me that I'd never practise Judo again, which as you can imagine, I found of little use. A chance meeting with a therapist a few weeks later whilst on holiday provided me with just the advice I needed for rehabilitation and some bodywork to relieve my screaming muscles of their tension.

Then one day, several years later, I found I had "golfer's elbow" - never touched a golf club in my life! It was a consequence of too much laptop work without regard to proper posture and ergonomic workstations - did you know that this condition is prevalent in work groups that are under stress or constant change and notice of redundancy? This lasted for 2 years. I couldn't pick up my toddlers without pain. I had physio, friction massage (boy did that bring tears to the eyes...even now as I remember and type about it) and the dreaded cortisone injections but nothing changed. Then one day, at a dance class, I met a lady who eyed the cuffs on my elbows with suspicion and told me that she could sort them - the elbows, not the cuffs.

Three sessions later and they were pain free! But that wasn't what impressed me. No, for 20 years I'd had a longstanding hip/sacro-iliac pain caused by too many landings in Judo and I'd learned to ignore it and cope. Well, it disappeared after the first session, and I hadn't even mentioned it to Nicola...I was impressed! But it would still be another 5 years before I decided to train as a Bowen therapist.

My work background is in research and development into advanced software engineering techniques such as artificial intelligence, virtual reality and genetic algorithms. For a time, I was also quite well known in the field of Human Computer Interaction and cognitive science. Being able to prove or disprove hypotheses, set up experiments, analyse the results, draw conclusions, and so on, were all very common day-to-day activities for me. So, I found it very interesting that the Bowen technique achieved remarkable results without really knowing why it did so (at that time). However, the same could be said of neural networks as well, but that didn't stop the investment in their practical applications. Perhaps because I had the R&D mentality, I was quite willing to accept such results without the need to know why...necessarily.

Musings of a Therapist

During the next 5-year period, I qualified as a Neuro-Linguistic Programming practitioner. That's basically concerned with understanding how people think, speak, and act. I applied this to my work as a telecomms consultant and also in my work as a Judo coach for children. My work also led me to become certified in health and safety and in particular in ergonomics. Then one day I found it was time to qualify as a Bowen therapist and I now practise part-time whilst continuing to be a consultant. I find the Bowen work to be extremely rewarding.

What's the point in all these ramblings? Well, I guess, it's to show you how my path into complementary therapies has influenced my thinking and feelings about practising complementary techniques and to show my qualifications and to be able to talk about certain subjects, such as business cases, which I do later.

So, there you have it, some of my qualifications and experience to talk about business activities, design a model to help classify therapies, comment on the abstract and ground in specifics.

Section 1

PRACTICALITIES OF BEING A THERAPIST

Introduction

I've attended several continuous professional development (CPD) courses for Bowen now, either as an assistant to the instructor or as a participant, and it still amazes me that there are so many people who have no idea whether they can make a living out of their chosen therapy. Instead they have a well-intentioned desire to "do good" and believe that, once they've trained, people will flock to them to be healed...only to be amazed when that doesn't happen. One year down the line they're on another course in the latest craze and no longer put into practice what they've already learned. Of course, there are those, like me, who want to do it part-time, or only intend to do friends and family, and that's fine.

Quite simply a lack of a business plan will lead to

despondency and despair. Or as the saying goes, a failure to plan is a plan to fail.

I don't intend to present an in-depth business plan generation piece here. There are lots of books and articles on this subject. If you're already a therapist then I'm sure you've done your homework. For those of you who are considering whether to start a therapy business then I include here some general things to consider and reading material references.

Similarly, I'm not going to discuss tax, law, or insurance, other than to say that you need to understand how they all apply to your situation. Most countries' government body now recognise that it's better to educate a person on how to fill in tax forms and set up businesses than it is to chase people for debt or take them through the legal system. Therefore, go and talk to your local government agencies for advice on what you want to do. They'll run courses on these topics for people in the same situation as yourself, and perhaps even more important, these people on your courses will form part of your personal business network.

Business Plan - Can I afford to be a Therapist?

Definition: A business plan is a written document that describes the nature of your business, your sales and marketing strategy, your financial background, along with a projected profit and loss statement.

A business plan is not just for you to convince a bank manager to lend you money, it's there to allow you to make decisions on how and where you want to practice, how long you will need to depend on the support and generosity of others, and so on. It reminds you where you're going once you've started to practice and helps you to make decisions for the good of your business.

In short it will define where you want your business to

be within a certain period of time (usually five years) and how you plan on getting there. Time spent putting together your plan together will be repaid several-fold over the next few years and will make your business decisions easier too.

In general, a business plan document contains the following material:

- Executive Summary
- Description of Business
- Description of your service (or product)
- Market Analysis
- Competitive Analysis
- Operations and Management
- Strategy and Implementation
- Financial Components
- Income Statement
- Cash Flow Statement
- Balance Sheet
- Projected Growth
- Supporting Documents

Anything else relevant to your plan such as client

references, copy of lease, etc.

There are three essential attributes to a good plan:

1) Specific milestones, assumptions, and tasks. Think of the 6 Ws - What, Where, When, How, Why, Who. What's the task? Why is it necessary? Who's going to do it? By When will it be done? How will it be achieved? Where will it take place?
2) Cash flow month by month. It's no use being profitable if you can't pay your bills.
3) Priorities. Don't try to do everything and don't try to please everyone!

The topics above should be quite self-explanatory. My references at the end of this book will point you to other useful information sources.

Remember: Failure to plan is to plan to fail.

How much should I charge?

As part of your business plan you'll need to work out how much you will charge for your sessions for instance. You'll need to look at what your competitors charge to get some idea of the market rates, and then you'll need to decide what you will charge. This will depend on how you brand yourself - cheap and cheerful vs. luxurious and valuable - and of course how much you need to earn. Here are some tips for you to consider.

Rules of Thumb

In general, there are approximately 200-240 working days in a year, or about 1,600 to 2,000 working hours. These figures assume that the rest of the time you're on holiday, sick, doing the books, reading, marketing, attending courses, etc. To keep sums simple, I choose 200 working days and 2,000 hours. This means that I can turn day and hourly rates into an annual figure quite easily.

For instance:

- $20 per hour = $40,000 annual income
- £300 per day = £60,000 annual income

So, if you intend to charge your clients $30 a session and a session is one hour long then, assuming that you can fill up every hour of your 8-hour working day, you'll earn about $60,000 a year. Of course, that's a big assumption, especially in the complementary therapy market! And did I say that this doesn't include breaks?!

Now, you also need to work out how much you need to earn to cover all your costs and leave you with money to spend. When you are in a full time company job, the salary you earn is only part of the overall package that the company spends on you. The package includes money for your holidays, pension, medical etc. The following table provides you with a list of some items against which you can allocate a cost and therefore come up with an annual monetary value that indicates how much you need to earn to enjoy the lifestyle you want. You'll notice that it doesn't include items such as marketing, rent, supplies, food, clothes, mortgage etc. You'll need to add these in as well. As a general rule, if you need to spend money on something put it in, no matter how small a cost it is.

ITEM	ANNUAL VALUE ($)
Holidays	2,000
Car Running Costs	5,000
Pension Contributions	2,000
Dental Contributions	400
Family Medical Insurance	400
Phone	240
Training	2,000
Professional Body Memberships	150
Accident Insurance	100
Etc.	
Total	**$12,290**

Another rule of thumb is that taxes account for about half of your annual earnings. So you would need to earn about $25,000 to ensure that you could take home $12,290.

$25,000 is equivalent to $125 per day.

Now you can start to see how much you need to charge your client and how many clients you need each day.

What's my Brand?

There are many therapies and therapists in any given town, so how do you make yourself stand out from the crowd and get people to come to you? This is perhaps the most important question to answer for your business plan. If you have no idea who you are and what you have to offer, why should anyone decide to come to you for relief?

Most therapists work in isolation, i.e. they are one-man bands. Even when they are part of a health centre that has other therapists this is often just a federation rather than a united company. So effectively, a therapist is selling themselves. And it's difficult to sell yourself, isn't it?

Musings of a Therapist

Recently, I read two books that provided some answers on how to do this effectively. The first is by Martin Fisher in his book "Now Pick Me!" On the face of it, his book is about how to get a job...but isn't this just what you want to do? And the second is "The Pitching Bible" by Paul Boross. Once you've read these books, I believe you will have the tools to answer the question, "How do you make yourself stand out from the crowd and get people to come to you?"

Fisher's book considers: "How to differentiate yourself from others with the same skills and experience." and Boross' book shows you how to convince people to choose you.

Once you've worked out the answer for your business, make sure that you always have two things with you:

- Your business cards: business cards are made to be given away, always.

- Your "elevator pitch": when someone asks you what you do, you need to be able to tell them in less than 30 seconds.

I think that business cards are self-explanatory but the elevator pitch requires a little more thought. When you ask someone what they do, how often do they reply with their job title or provide the name of their company or market sector? E.g. "I'm an Accountant", or "I work in telecommunications"? These aren't particularly informative or interesting, are they?

Wouldn't it be more interesting and informative to say something like:

- "I help people save money by showing them how to fill in their tax forms properly."
- "I ensure that people can send texts to each other by keeping the network running."

So, your elevator pitch needs to tell them in one sentence, what benefit you bring them and how you do it. If the person is interested, then you'll get the "tell me more" signal, which then gives you the opportunity to spend the other 25 seconds telling them a little more. The purpose of the pitch is to get enough of their interest that they'll ask your advice, ask you for more information, or even better, make an appointment to see you.

Here are some example conversations for you. Tell me which turns you off and which piques your interest:

Conversation 1:

"What do I do?"

"Well, I'm a Bowen Practitioner"

"What's Bowen and how does it work?

"Bowen is a technique that uses a gentle rolling action over muscles, tendons, ligaments that causes the muscles to relax. Once they relax the body resets its healing mechanism and addresses all the problems with the body, deciding which ones to sort out first. The moves must be carried out in a precise sequence. It's very gentle and I also leave the room for a few minutes to give the body time to work out what it's going to do."

Conversation 2:

"What do I do?"

"I help people to get better"

"Really, how do you do that?"

"By using my fingers to help their bodies relax and encourage their own healing mechanisms to fix their own problems."

"Wow, that sounds simple, how does that work"

"It is simple and it works really well. Even better, it's very gentle and non-invasive. Here's my card, ring the number, make an appointment and you can see for yourself how effective it is."

Well, I hope you went for the second conversation. The difference is that in the second one I'm telling them the benefits of what I do. If instead I describe how it works as in the first conversation, two things will happen:

1. They'll want to equate it to something they know like Osteopathy for instance and therefore apply their own expectations to how it will work.

2. They won't figure out how it will benefit them and therefore lose interest.

Once you've worked out the answers to "how do you make yourself stand out from the crowd and get people to come to you?", they will form the basis of your marketing and advertising campaign and appear in some form on your business cards, leaflets, banners and any other promotional items.

Advertising

Many therapists seem to think that just because they're trained in a complementary therapy, the world will beat a path to their door. And when they don't, they can't understand why and become disenchanted and blame it on the therapy. Or perhaps the thought of marketing oneself is rather too much like blowing one's own trumpet. Others know that to be a success they have to become known but don't how to become known.

For every therapist you ask you'll get a different answer to the question of what marketing activities work best. Why is it that one says that leafleting brings in several clients yet another will say that they've never had a response to a leaflet through the door? Personally, I don't know! Perhaps the successful leaflet person designed a good leaflet, or the people who received the leaflets preferred leaflets to radio adverts, or the leaflet person had a conversation with someone in the household. Suffice to say that you'll only find out when you try it yourself.

However, I do think that there are some thoughts to bear in mind about how people communicate with each other. Every person, including you, has a preferred method of taking in information. The main ways are:

- Visually - something they see
- Auditory - something they hear
- Kinaesthetic - something they feel
- Digital - something that causes them to think

If you communicate with someone using their preferred method of communication they are more likely to hear what you're saying, or perhaps see what you're saying, or even feel what you're saying! This doesn't mean that the only way to communicate effectively with auditory people is to advertise on the radio. No, what it means is that you have to use words or language that fit into these categories. As an example, let's assume that someone describes a problem to you with their shoulder. You might respond with something like:

- Yes, I see that it causes you pain
- Yes, I can tell that's painful
- Yes, that would hurt
- Yes, that makes sense that that would be painful

The trick is to be able to detect what communication style is best for your client.

But what's this got to do with marketing? Well, it means that different marketing methods work for different people and that for each marketing method you have to use words that appeal to as many types of people as possible. Let's take a leaflet for example. You can make it visually appealing - colours, pictures, layout etc. you can make it kinaesthetic through the type of paper used, does it feel nice, does it feel like quality? But how to appeal to auditory or digital people? This would have to be considered in the words used in the leaflet. For example, "can you afford time off work because of your shoulder injury?" - digital/logical.

Musings of a Therapist

"If I told you, you could have a sound shoulder in only 2 weeks by calling me now..." - auditory. If it was a radio advert...imagine how you would feel...

Those of you who are familiar with Neuro-Linguistic Programming will recognise what I'm saying here. For those who aren't, my references at the end of the book contain some introductions to NLP that are well worth reading.

Get out and about

Sounds simple really and it is but that doesn't mean it's easy to do. You will need to spend a lot of time getting to know your area and for your area to get to know you. Marketing isn't a one-off activity. It's something you need to do every day. You should set aside around 10% of each day to engage in marketing-type activities and at least once a month where you spend half-a-day or more at public events.

Daily marketing activities include:

- Updating your web-site/blog
- Writing to your clients' doctors
- Talking to prospective clients
- Putting up notices in shop windows

- Creating your leaflets
- Giving away your business cards

Monthly Activities include:

- Presenting to your local Business club, Women's Institute, etc.
- Giving demonstrations in a shopping centre
- Attending an exhibition
- Writing an article for your local newspaper
- Giving an interview on local radio

You should never be bored when you don't have clients on your couch!

Where to Practise?

Where you want to practise your therapy depends to a large extent on your type of personality. Are you self-motivating or do you need to work with others? Are you good at selling yourself or do you need someone to do this for you? I believe there are three ways of working, each with its own advantages and disadvantages.

1. In a Practice or Health Care Centre

Becoming part of a centre that accommodates other therapists has many advantages:

- Rooms are provided
- Appointments are booked on your behalf
- Other therapists are available to chat with

- The premises are safe and secure
- The place looks professional
- Marketing and branding is in place
- Your personal safety

For me, this is the ideal way for a therapist just starting out in business or those doing it part-time. The established infrastructure allows you to concentrate solely on the therapy you provide and to build up your client base.

There are disadvantages:

- You have to pay rent
- You can't change the way the room looks
- The opinions of the other therapists on how to run the centre have to be taken into account

But overall, it relieves you of a lot of pressure and allows you to find out in a safe way whether the market likes you and your therapy and more importantly whether you like this job.

2. At home

Working from home has a number of things to consider. First and foremost is will it look professional? To look professional, I think that there needs to be a room that is dedicated to the therapy, has space to move around the couch, is safe, and is welcoming yet devoid of personal belongings. And the preference is for that room to be separated from the rest of the house, either by way of another entrance or is an annexe to the house.

Such an environment shows that you are serious about your business, professional in your attitude, and sets up the proper boundaries for a client-therapist relationship. It also means you focus properly and you both know that you are there to discuss matters related to the client and the therapy rather than pleasant social chit chat leading to a perceived friendship.

As well as concentrating on your therapy, you also need to allocate time to marketing, sales, ordering stock and so on. You might well find yourself spending more time on these aspects than on the therapy you enjoy.

Working from home works for me if it's for people I know well, friends, family, and long standing clients.

3. At people's homes

Practising at the client's home is fraught with problems and yet is sometimes unavoidable. I only do this if I know the person well or they have been to my clinic for a few sessions. If you're just starting out in this business, I would avoid it completely until you are very confident of your skills and reading of potentially unsafe situations. Unsafe doesn't just mean from personal, physical attacks but from other situations such as allegations of stealing, molestation, and hurting yourself through poor posture brought on by poorly positioned couches or beds.

Note Taking

You **must** take notes before, during, and after your sessions. And you need these for a variety of reasons:

- history taking on the first session;
- before each session to find out what happened to your client immediately after the last session and in the time between the last one and now;
- during the session to record observations by both you and your client;
- To enable you to compare the progress of your client from session to session (see leading the witness).

And what is **extremely important**, is to make sure that you can defend yourself in case of any litigations against you that are brought on by your client claiming malpractice!

What this means is that your notes need to be understandable and allow you to slip back into the context of the session several years later. Whilst the law varies from country to country, you will need to keep your notes for several years, in a secured place. Should you be taken to court, the only defence you have are your notes. And your defence will only be as good as your notes!

In the UK, notes need to be kept for a minimum of 5 years because a client can claim within 3 years of the session if they think that you injured them or made them worse. However, that limit only applies when the client is over 18 years of age. If they are 12 years old now, they can start the claim when they are between 18 and 21 years of age. So in this case your notes would need to be kept for up to 16 years!

The best way to take notes is entirely a personal

preference; there is no right or wrong way...just an "are they detailed and understandable enough to defend you several years later?" way.

I've tried several ways to take notes ranging from computer-based form filling to hand written free form. The latter currently works best for me as I like to draw diagrams and lines joining notes from different session. I use an A4 piece of paper in landscape mode so I can note down a few columns of sessions on each side. I also draw a timeline of each client upon which I note various incidents throughout their lifetime.

In the future, I'll move to a computer tablet once they're able to accurately and quickly record my pen marks.

Section 2

A THERAPIST MODEL

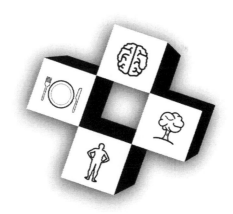

Dave Riches

Introduction

For a long time, I had a model that described what was required to make and keep a body healthy and sound. It had 3 aspects to it, which was really nice because it could be described quite succinctly in a diagram such as a triangle that showed them all in balance. The 3 aspects were: Physical, Mental, and Environment. If you want to change the body, you have to change the way the person thinks about the body and you have to change the environment within which the physical problems have occurred. For example, Repetitive Strain. Doesn't it make sense that if the cause of the strain is not removed then healing the strain only solves part of the problem? Likewise, if the person believes that every time they make a move it will cause pain, then it will.

This was all quite sensible. Then, as I started to get older and my body didn't recover quickly enough from the stresses of Judo and dancing, it didn't matter whether my mind was right (mental), my throwing technique was right (environment), my body was fixable (physical), it just took too long. This was when it became obvious, to me at least, that my model was wrong or needed to be enhanced. And that's when I took an interest in Nutrition. It was now blindingly obvious that if your body doesn't have the resources, the bricks and mortar, to rebuild the body then all the good intentions of treating the physical, mental, and environmental aspects would eventually be for naught, or at the very least, take longer to resolve.

So now my model has 4 parts to it:

- **Physical wellbeing** - how do I correct the physical layout of the body?
- **Mental wellbeing** - how do I think, speak, feel, and act about my problem?
- **Inner wellbeing (nutrition)** - has my body got the building blocks to repair the damage?
- **Environment -** do my work, home, and social environments allow me to get better?

As a therapist, I believe that all these aspects need to be considered during the development of a programme for the client to get better. Have a look at my musings on this. It might be the case that they come thinking that a physical intervention is required when in fact you conclude that a mental intervention would be better. If you're not trained in mental interventions then you would refer them to a practitioner who does.

Physical Wellbeing

Insert here your favourite physical intervention - massage, osteopathy, manipulation, etc. Mine of course is the Bowen Technique. Developed in Australia by Tom Bowen during the mid-1900s it is a very effective technique. Characterised by slow, gentle movements over muscles, ligaments and tendons, with long waits between movements, the technique encourages the fascia of the body to return to an efficient and effective state, which promotes the wellbeing of the body across the hormonal, nervous, and musculo-skeletal systems. There are several good books on this bodywork technique, and training courses are readily available.

I am so pleased with the results that I achieve with the Bowen Technique that I do not feel the need to add to my toolkit in this area. That's not to say that I won't in the future but for now I'm content.

Mental Wellbeing

Again, you could insert your favourite method to address the way in which people think, speak and feel about their problems. I'm not a fan of methods that require the client to recount troubled times over and over again as I believe that this just reinforces the problem. I favour those that promote a forward-looking, positive intent that move the client from a state where they have little control (the victim) to one where they feel responsible for their own self. You might have guessed that my preferred technique is through NLP (Neuro-Linguistic Programming) interventions. Others might favour CBT (Cognitive Behavioural Therapy) or EFT (Emotional Freedom Technique). And again, for where I am now, I am quite content with NLP as my tool, or rather set of tools for this aspect of my model. Some references to good NLP books are provided later.

Inner Wellbeing - Nutrition

Now that I've spent more time talking to Nutritionists and reading up on this area it seems so obvious to me that this needs to be a fundamental part of education at primary schools and above. I took A-Level Human Biology many years ago and more recently Anatomy & Physiology as part of my Bowen accreditation. Just revisiting and reminding me of how the body works showed how much of what is held to be "general knowledge" about food today is just rubbish. Instead it shows me how powerful the marketing machine is.

As a starting point, I'd highly recommend a documentary shown on the BBC in 2012 - "The Men who made us Fat" and the works of Dr Paul Clayton, "Health Defence". If they don't inspire you to take a closer look at what you put into your body then I don't know what will. At the very least, reduce your sugar and gluten intake.

Dave Riches

The following is taken from an article on the results of a study into the importance of breakfast for school students. You'll notice that there's more than just nutrition to consider, such as the stigma of eating free breakfasts. The article reference is: Nathan Greenfield; "The view from here - Canada – Behaviour improvement in the best possible taste"; Published in TES magazine on 18 November, 2011.

Following the 2007 shooting of a 15-year-old boy in a high school in a poor and violent part of Toronto, many expected principals to call for a US-style crackdown. But instead of hardening their schools with metal detectors and extra police, school leaders told the city's board of education that the best way to improve morale, behaviour and school performance was to feed pupils breakfast and lunch.

After three years, the programme showed some astounding results. Prior to the programme, 68% of students came to school having had no breakfast; and 20% missed both breakfast and lunch!

Now that breakfast and lunch are available to

everyone, scores have improved substantially across the board in reading and science; and the number of 15-year-olds graduating is significantly higher when compared to those who miss breakfast and lunch. Emotional behaviour has also improved. "If a child has poor problem-solving and conflict-resolution skills, he or she is more likely to be a behaviour problem," the teacher said. "Students in the programme score higher on conflict-resolution and problem-solving tests." These differences show up in their behaviour in class and even in suspensions and expulsions, which dropped by half."

"We started by putting food out in the hallway thinking that hungry kids would take it, but they wouldn't because of the stigma," said the teacher. "So we opted to feed every child every day."

The food programme started as a creative response to a tragic shooting. But with the results in, it could lead to fewer children across the country missing meals and the chance of educational success.

There are many stories like this that serve to show the importance of good, nutritional meals.

Environment

The environment covers personal and work places, and both the physical and social aspects. The workplace is well covered by Health and Safety regulations, perhaps too much some might say. However, the ergonomics of how you should sit or stand at work seem to be less well known despite there being regulations in place. With many jobs requiring computer work these days, much research has gone into defining what is the best layout of monitor, keyboard, telephone, lighting, chair etc. but few take the time to adjust their workplace until they've suffered a repetitive strain injury. Every business has a duty of care to educate its workforce on how to sit, how to lift, and how to avoid injury at work.

And then there's your home or place of rest, do you take as much care of this physical environment as you do (or should) your work environment? When you lift your child up, do you bend your knees? When you reach for something high up in the cupboard what do you stand on? Do you leave toys or clothes at the top of the stairs?

The social aspect is often more insidious and harder to change. If you client returns home to a bullying environment will their wellbeing continue to improve after your intervention? If their company is laying off lots of people will their RSI get better? I'd say that there is little that you can do here other than educate your client on what types of environment are conducive to wellbeing. They have to make the decision on how to change their social environment. But you can give them the tools to help them make those decisions and how to change the way they react to their social environment.

An Example

Some time ago I wrote an article entitled "Why won't they lie still and stop talking?" in which I discussed what it meant to be a practitioner and outlined my therapist model described earlier. The following is a description of how someone came to me because they thought the Bowen would help but in fact it wasn't required because it was addressed by one of the other parts of my model, the Mental aspect.

The Client

A friend of my daughter was experiencing severe headaches several times a day at school. At the school gates I discussed the possibility with her mother of having some Bowen therapy. Her mum decided to give it a try because she was very concerned about the long term effect the headaches were having on her daughter, tiredness, irritability and so on. At the time, the daughter, Linda, was 8 years old. She was a shy and timid girl in large company but quite fun and jolly in small groups; and she was quite small for her age.

The Session

Linda came round one evening after school with her mother. I sat her on my couch and sat myself next to the couch on a lower level. Her mother remained in the room throughout and Linda was quite comfortable talking to me. I asked Linda the usual background information about her health and previous accidents, and then moved on to the subject of headaches. Here she became a little reticent and responded a "don't know" to most of the questions – no, she didn't know why she got headaches, nor the reasons they occurred at similar times throughout the day.

I decided to change the style of my questions and

asked her to ask her body how it knew it was time to have a headache...and got that look that children give when they're think you're teasing but aren't sure! What's the matter, I asked, don't you talk to your body? No? But your body talks to you, don't you listen to it? So I explained how the body talks in different ways and told her that if she listened she'd hear it talking.

Once she had decided that she could hear her body talk to her things moved along nicely. She remembered a time when she had a headache and she told me its sub-modalities - its colour, shape, size, mass, temperature, place in body etc. Then I asked her to remember a time when she felt calm and happy, and elicited the sub-modalities again. Shape and colour were the major differences and I showed her how to change each of them from the migraine values to the calm and happy values.

When she found it easy to make the changes, which in children is usually quite quick, I then asked her to foresee a time in the future when she was at school and her body was telling her it was time to have a headache...and told her to make the changes, which she did. She looked at me excitedly and smiled happily at the ease with which she could make and feel the change.

The end...or perhaps the beginning?

I didn't see her for several weeks as I wasn't picking up the kids for a while. I bumped into her and her mum in town one day and I asked how she was doing at school. Any headaches? Oh no, I don't get those any more, she said airily, if my body says it's time, I just change the colour and it goes away! I just love this stuff!

I could have used Bowen but it didn't seem appropriate or necessary. Instead, I gave her a tool to help her remain calm and be able to think clearly in times of stress. The tool gave her the resource to change her body, mind, and view of her environment. I'd like to think that she still remembers how to use it several years later but who knows?

Section 3

MUSINGS

Why Won't They Lie Still and Stop Talking?

Have you ever had the person who comes in to your clinic and talks and talks and talks? You've only an hour per session and already 10 minutes have gone by. Surely this person came for some Bowen to get better...and they haven't even mentioned what the problem is yet! Or have they?

Or perhaps, a client returns every 3 months or so with the same problem each time. Surely I sorted that in the first couple of sessions, why are they back again, I thought this Bowen technique got to the root of the problem not just its symptoms?

But maybe, just maybe, the "problem" is me, the

therapist? Maybe I'm not listening properly; maybe I'm too keen to start the Bowen so that I can help the person get better; maybe I think the answer always is Bowen...now, what was the question?

I'm a Bowen therapist; do I need to perform Bowen to help the person get better?

Do you remember the last time you went to a therapist, a doctor, a dentist? How did you feel about the visit? Were your concerns addressed to your satisfaction? If not, why not? If yes, what was it about your visit that helped you?

Take some time to think about how it feels to be a client...what makes you feel better? Sometimes it's simply because someone listened. Sometimes it's a change in your physical activity. Sometimes it's a change of your normal diet. Sometimes it's making a change in your environment. Sometimes it's because you were made to look at something in a different way. Sometimes it's a bit of healing. So any one, some, or all of these changes might help your client to feel better.

As a practitioner we need to make sure that they're all

considered in our programme to help a client get better. To help me make sure I've considered more than just the Bowen aspect, I've divided them into the following considerations:

1) Mental wellbeing
2) Physical wellbeing
3) The Environment within which the client moves/lives
4) Internal wellbeing – Nutrition

Each one needs to be explored during a session with the client. Sometimes, the mere fact that the clients vocalise what's happening in their lives in each of these areas is enough to start the healing process.

So, just because I'm a Bowen practitioner does that mean that people come to me so that I can perform Bowen on them, or do they come to me because they want to get better? If the latter, then if I explore the considerations above do I need to do any Bowen during the session? I know what my answers are, what are yours?

Helping the Client to see Progress

Client: "I'm not getting better, I haven't noticed any change!"

How often do you get a client who says nothing happened during the session or during the week before the next session but you can see the change, and so can others? So, what's happening or more importantly, how can you make them notice the change in themselves?

Musings of a Therapist

Q: "Why should I care if they don't notice, I know the Bowen is working and they are getting better?"

It's important that the client notices the change for two reasons:

1) It promotes a positive mental attitude that allows further change to be received positively and progress to be made more quickly.

2) The client believes that Bowen works and therefore promotes it (and returns for a further session).

Q: "How do I help them notice change then?"

You have 3 opportunities to help them notice the change:

1) During your history taking when you establish a baseline of measurable events.

2) During your sessions with your use of language patterns.

3) During your follow-up at the beginning of the next session by highlighting changes to the events elicited in (1) above.

Q: "Could you explain further and provide me with some examples?"

Sure, let's take them one at time:

Elicitation of Measurable Events

Taking the history of the client has several purposes including: an understanding of how the current condition came about; whether there are other conditions that might interact with the current one; are there things in the past that contribute to the current condition and so on. Whilst these are of interest, the most important one is to establish a baseline of the number of times an event occurs even if that event doesn't appear to be a contributing factor to the current condition of the client.

From this baseline, it then becomes easy to determine whether the frequency of occurrence for each event has changed from session to session.

Q: "How do I spot a measurable event?"

Well, this comes from the way in which you ask your questions, and of course becomes easier with practice. Usually, the client will make a comment that includes an adverb – adverbs tells us when, how or where something happens. Words ending in –ly are commonly adverbs but not always. As an example, "I frequently go to the toilet during the night."; "I usually wake up with an aching back."; "I often get these dizzy spells."

Your job is to spot these generalisations and ask the client to be specific. "How frequently do you go the toilet?"; "How many times during the week do you wake up with an aching back?"; "When you say often, how often do you mean?" You note the answers and refer to them in the next session.

To get to this stage, where the client is able to provide you with clues to identify metrics, you need to have asked open questions such as, "Tell me about..."; "Describe what happened when..." These provide the opportunity for the client to spend time talking (please let them) and for you to spot the adverbs and ask the closed questions, "How often?", "At what time?" Make sure you don't interrupt the flow of the client too often, it's important that they feel that you have listened to their concerns.

Use of Language Patterns

Once you've finished your note taking, it's time for the session. There are three stages where you have the opportunity to prepare the client's mind to believe that change is inevitable:

>1) As part of the setup for the session, i.e. before your first set of moves.

For example, you might state, *"Experience shows that the majority of people experience sensations during the session, some might find a muscle starts to twitch; some might become hot or cold; others will tingle; to some it might be that part of the body feels...different. A very few might not notice anything and that's also ok."*

People don't like to feel left out, so the statement that the "majority" feels something is important. However, the last statement is just as important because we don't want to make them uneasy/worried if they don't notice anything. The intention here is to make their mind believe that change is a natural consequence of the therapy.

2) The Bowen 2-minute breaks.

"Whilst I'm out of the room, I want you to close your eyes and pay attention to your body. Notice what changes have happened no matter where they occur in your body nor how small they might be. When I come back, I will ask what you felt and your answers will enable me to decide which moves to perform on you."

Here the words act as a command for the client to notice something because they believe it's important to their wellbeing. Also, we want them to bring to our attention anything, no matter how small, rather than to dismiss that very small twitch as nothing of consequence.

3) Return for the next set of moves.

"Tell me what you noticed."

The wording is important. There is an implicit assumption here that something happened and the client feels a compulsion to think deeply about the response. Compare this with the statement, "Did you notice anything?" which is a closed question and easy to answer as "No." with little thought given to the question or the answer. I also find it important to ask them to be specific. For example, "The fingers in my left hand tingled." gets the response, "Which fingers?"

4) General comments.

I also ask whether the changes are still happening, whether they're getting more or less, and use the answers as an indication of whether or when to continue.

Sometimes the client asks whether a response is good or bad and in my opinion it's neither...just data. I do note though that any change is good change. The body is moving from its "stuck" state to a new state, and therefore that's good.

Some responses though have more obvious meanings and I refer you to the Mind Body Bowen Course run by Anne Spicer and Margaret Schubert for further development.

Noting the Changes

At the next session, you must begin with a review of how they felt the rest of the day after the session; and how they felt during the week. Finish this part of the session with a review of the metrics that you discovered the previous session. Make sure that you pick up on any new metrics to add to your baseline. The purpose of this is to make sure that your client is aware of changes to the baseline and therefore gain confidence that your therapy is working. This is also an opportunity to note changes in the body language and speech of the client.

You need to make sure that any changes have been noted by the client and re-inforced by your speech.

Q: "Well that's a lot to consider, what final comments do you have?"

Good Data and Language.

How somebody feels is extremely subjective. To influence their feeling we must present a case that is difficult to refute. That happens only with good data and consistent measurement of that data. Taking this further, for Bowen or any other alternative therapy to become accepted in the mainstream, we must have a multitude of good case references where change is obviously proven. You can create your own standard of metrics to ask about and record for analysis. I refer you to MYMOP - Measure yourself medical outcome profile – as a good starting place.

Language is extremely important, not just for how you speak to your clients but also to understand what it is they're not saying to you (but want you to find out!) NLP (Neuro-Linguistic Programming) is an excellent tool. If you're not aware of this technique, I refer you to "Principles of NLP - The Only Introduction You'll Ever Need" by Joseph O'Connor and Ian McDermott.

And finally, there are no difficult clients, only interesting ones. It's your responsibility to find them of interest and to help them to notice their progress to well-being.

Your Posture

The first rule of therapy, just like in First Aid, is to look after your own safety first. In particular, I'm referring to your posture whilst delivering your bodywork. However, there are of course other aspects such as, if you're using your home as your place of work, how do you make sure your client won't harm you, or stalk you later?

Why should posture matter? Well, consider these questions:

> 1) If your therapy is your living, can you afford to take time off from your business?

2) What will clients think if you're the one who hobbles or has bandages over your wrist, elbow, knee etc?

3) What use are you to your clients if you can't perform the procedures properly?

4) Can you practice if you're injured?

So you have to look after your own physical wellbeing first. I've divided this into two categories:

1) Your environment

2) Your posture

Your environment

As a matter of course, you need to perform a health and safety check or risk assessment of your work area to ensure that your client won't hurt themselves just by being in your work area. For instance, are there trip hazards, sharp corners on couches, water on the floor, etc?

Then there's your safety in the environment. Is there enough space around the couch for you to move without tripping? Is your couch set at the right height for you to work comfortably? When you reach for towels, tools of your trade, etc. do you have to stretch awkwardly or are they in easy reach?

Take time to design the layout of your work area so that everything is easy for you to do.

Your posture

Posture is everything. Poor posture leads to fatigue, injury, and poor application of your bodywork. Working several hours a day, performing similar movements, reaching for tools, helping people sit up or lie down, is a tiring business. When people get tired, mistakes creep in, technique suffers, and injuries occur. Make sure that:

- You stand up properly
- Your feet are in the right position, i.e. underneath you
- Don't reach outside your circle of gravity
- Your shoulder, arms, wrists, hands are

relaxed
- Protect your lower back
- Take regular breaks
- Drink lots of water
- Have another therapist give you a session

Just like dancers, martial artists, and sportsmen concentrate on technique and posture so you should too.

Towel Management

It might seem strange to muse about towel management but listen first to my story and then you'll see why. Picture this, newly qualified; I've found a place to practice in, first client walks in the door. She's young, just had a little boy, and speaks little English. I do my best; all my rehearsed introductions and explanations go out the window as I have to speak slowly, clearly, and as plainly as possible. I ask her to undress to her underwear and get on the couch. I leave the room, and wait a few minutes. I come back in to find she's mis-understood my instructions and is lying nude on the couch! Fortunately, she's lying prone, so my blushing and hesitancy goes unnoticed. Once the towels are placed on her, normal order is restored...for a while.

Musings of a Therapist

The session goes well, and then it's time to turn her over. Of course, she doesn't turn the way I expect her to and her lower half is briefly exposed. Then, at the end, it's time to sit her up. Already a little nervous from the first mishap, I put my arm round her shoulders to grab the other end of the towel but she's already moving to sit up and I miss the towel. And of course, as she does so, the towel slips off her top half and I fumble to pick it back up. Needless to say, she didn't come back for another session and never took up my future discount programmes!

Over the next few weeks, whilst I waited for the litigation letter to drop through the door, I practised with the towels, and now I believe I've got it right, even when performing the seated shoulder move. It's tricky to explain what I do without demonstration but let's try. In a session, I use 2 bath towels, one for the upper body and one for the waist down. The upper towel is laid across the body with the long side at right angles to the body; the lower towel is laid lengthwise down the body. There are 3 main times during a session when I pay particular attention to towel management:

Turning over

In the beginning, whenever I held up the towels to allow the client to turn over they would turn the opposite way to what I expected. The towels wouldn't keep them covered and would get caught up with their arms and legs. Even if I told them which way to turn, they'd go the other way! So now, I lift the towels by holding the far side of the body towel with both hands, one at the top corner and one at the bottom corner. My lower hand holds both the bottom corner of the body towel and the top corner of the leg towel. I then lean against the couch with my right leg to trap the top towel in place. When I raise the far side of the towels I then get a tight stretch on the towels between my leg and hands. So it doesn't matter how roughly the client turns over, the towels remain in place and the clients slides around underneath them. When they finish wriggling, the body towel is always in a perfect position when I lower it, and the leg towel needs just a little adjustment.

Sitting up

I need to make sure the body towel, especially, does not slip during the sitting up process. I do this by slipping my arm under their neck and shoulders and grabbing the top corner of the body towel. My other hand holds the top corner nearest to me. As I help them to sit up, I bring my hands together and use the farthest hand to grab both corners. So the towel now acts like a baby's bib, or barbers sheet. I then move my free hand to the leg towel to make sure that it doesn't fall off as they swing their legs to sit on the side of the couch.

I always have them sit on the side of the couch for a while as they'll often be a little dizzy after lying down for a period. I make sure that the hold I have on the top towel is firm, so that I can support them if they do start to keel over. When they're ready to stand up, I maintain that strong top grip for the same reason and hold the leg towel as it falls away so they don't trip over it.

I then walk them to a chair to sit down and maintain the top towel grip until they've sat down, where their body traps the towel against the back of the chair so there's no chance of it slipping down unexpectedly. Some people have a large peg that they use. I then replace the lower towel over their legs.

General rearrangement

I only re-arrange towels after the turn over. Other than that, I don't fuss over the towels. Some people tweak the towels every time they go by to make it look neat and tidy. When I have bodywork I find that quite annoying and it creates a draught. So unless the towels are in danger of falling off or showing a substantial portion of the body, I leave them alone.

In conclusion, the purpose of good towel management is to maintain the Dignity of the client and avoid the embarrassment of both the client and the practitioner.

Too Many Tools

I've met many therapists during my Bowen training, continuous professional development modules, and other events. All of them want to help make people better. Some of them believe that the way to do this is to learn as may therapies as possible, and all of them in the physical wellbeing field. Personally, I feel that rather than learning many therapies in one area, it's better to learn one well within each of the aspects of my therapy model, i.e. one in physical, one in mental, etc. Or, as I have done, be part of a health centres where there are experts in each of the aspects and refer clients to each other as appropriate.

Case Study Creation

If complementary therapies are to become accepted by mainstream medical professions and by insurance companies then we need to provide more empirical evidence of their usefulness. Where possible they need to be rigorous but for the likes of the ordinary practitioner this is unlikely to be practical. However, it is quite easy to set up an informal case study with a number of metrics to be measured. The more of these types of studies that are performed the more likely it will be that more formal studies will be sponsored to provide the rigour demanded by the core medical profession. And in turn, for complementary therapies to become part of mainstream client wellness programmes.

There are a couple of evaluation methods, and several

physical measurement tools, available to help record changes in client wellbeing.

Evaluation Methods

MYMOP (Measure Yourself Medical Outcome Profile) sometimes known as MYMOP2 as in the 2nd version.
http://sites.pcmd.ac.uk/mymop/index.php?c=intro

MYMOP is a client-generated, or individualised, outcome questionnaire. It is problem-specific but includes general wellbeing. It is applicable to all clients who present with symptoms, and these can be physical, emotional or social. It is brief and simple to administer.

COPM (Canadian Occupational Performance Measure)
https://www.caot.ca/copm/

COPM© is an individualized outcome measure designed for use by occupational therapists. The measure is designed to detect change in a client's self-perception of occupational performance over time.

Either of these evaluation methods is fine to use. Just choose the one that most suits you and look within your professional organisations for others that do the same and/or a repository where you can store your studies and look up other studies performed by other practitioners in your therapy.

Section 4

And Finally...

I do hope that you have found something to interest you or to spark off some thoughts on how to practice. If you would like to discuss any of my material or to suggest improvements, you can reach me at:

dave.riches@bowen-technique.co.uk

Bibliography

I have found the following sources of information to be very valuable in my quest to become a good therapist and to be able to support my model for a therapist. Some of these are referenced in my Musings and the rest are there for your enjoyment. Some of the references are specific to the UK however i) there is an equivalent for your country; and, ii) it's still useful to know ☺

Ref.	Author(s)	Title
1	Martin Fisher	"Now Pick Me!: A practical guide for being picked for the job you want"
2	Paul Boross	The Pitching Bible: The Seven Secrets of a Successful Business Pitch
3	Dr Paul Clayton	Health Defence
4	Ed Conduit	The Body Under Stress: Developing Skills for Keeping Healthy
5	Thomas W. Myers	"Anatomy Trains: Myofascial Meridians for Manual and Movement Therapists"

6	F. Batmanghelidj	"Your Body's Many Cries for Water: You're Not Sick; You're Thirsty: Don't Treat Thirst with Medications"
7	National Academic Press	"Dietary Reference Intakes for Water, Potassium, Sodium, Chloride, Sulfate"
8	Andrew Biel	Trail Guide to the Body
9	Andrew Matthews	"Being Happy – A Handbook to Greater Confidence and Security".
10	Isabel Briggs Myers	Gifts Differing: Understanding Personality Type
11	J O'Connor & Ian McDermott	Principles of NLP: The Only Introduction You'll Ever Need
12	H.M.R.C.	Business and Self-Employed, https://www.gov.uk/browse/business
13	UK Health & Safety	Health & Safety in the Workplace, http://www.hse.gov.uk/risk/
14	Ergonomics in Australia	How to Sit at a Computer, http://www.ergonomics.com.au

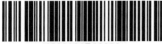

Printed in Great Britain
by Amazon.co.uk, Ltd.,
Marston Gate.